The Super-Fast Keto Vegan Recipe Book

Easy, Fast and Vegan Recipes for a Balanced Lifestyle

Karen Yosco

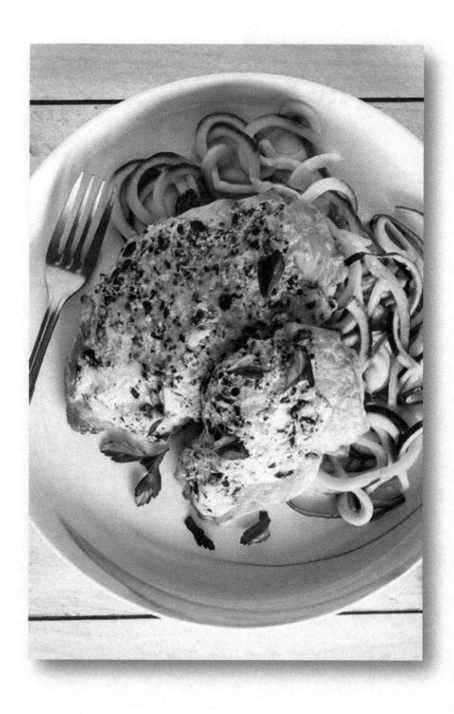

Table of Contents

BREAKFAST

Carrot Cake Oats

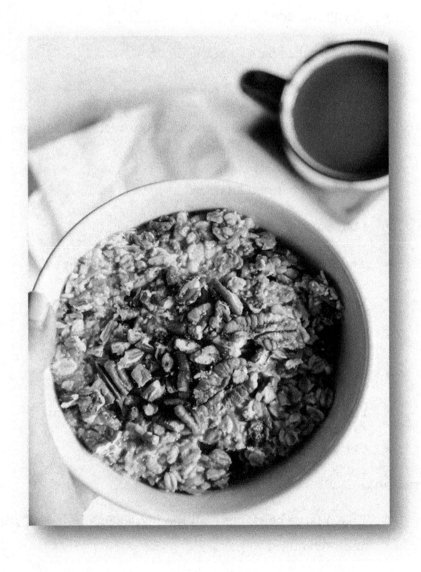

Preparation Time: 6 hours and 10 minutes

Cooking Time: 0 minutes

Servings: 4

Ingredients:

- ¼ cup shredded carrot

- 1/3 cup rolled oats

- 2 tablespoons chopped pineapple

- 1 tablespoon shredded coconut, unsweetened and more for topping

- 1 tablespoon ground flaxseed

- 1 tablespoon raisins and more for topping

- 2 tablespoons maple syrup and more for topping

- 1/8 teaspoon ground nutmeg

- ¼ teaspoon ground cinnamon and more for topping

- ¼ teaspoon vanilla extract, unsweetened

- 1 tablespoon chopped walnuts and more for topping

- ½ cup almond milk, unsweetened

Directions:

1. Take a large bowl, place all the ingredients in it, and stir until well mixed.

2. Cover the bowl with lid, and then place it in the refrigerator for a minimum of a minimum of 6 hours.

3. When ready to eat, distribute oats mixture evenly among 4 bowls, top with some shredded coconut, raisins, and walnuts, sprinkle with cinnamon, drizzle with maple syrup and then serve.

Nutrition: 242 Cal 9 g Fat 2 g Saturated Fat 35 g Carbohydrates 6 g Fiber 12 g Sugars 7 g Protein

Chocolate Chip and Coconut Pancakes

Preparation Time: 10 minutes

Cooking Time: 40 minutes

Servings: 8

Ingredients:

- 1¼ cups buckwheat flour

- 1 tablespoon flaxseeds

- 2 tablespoons coconut flakes, unsweetened

- ¼ cup rolled oats

- 1/8 teaspoon sea salt

- 1 tablespoon baking powder

- 1/3 cup mini chocolate chips, vegan

- ¼ cup maple syrup

- 1 teaspoon vanilla extract, unsweetened

- ½ cup applesauce, unsweetened

- 1 cup almond milk, unsweetened

- ½ cup of water

- 2 bananas, peeled, sliced

Directions:

1. Take a small saucepan, place it over medium heat, add flaxseeds, pour in water, and then cook for 4 to 5 minutes until sticky mixture comes together.

2. Strain the flaxseeds mixture immediately into a cup, discard the seeds, and set aside the collected flax water until required.

3. Take a large bowl, add buckwheat flour and oats in it, and then stir in salt, baking powder, and coconut until mixed.

4. Take a medium bowl, add 2 tablespoons of reserved flax water along with maple syrup and vanilla, pour in applesauce and milk, and whisk until combined.

5. Pour the milk mixture into the flour mixture, whisk well until thick batter comes together, and then fold in chocolate chips.

6. Take a griddle pan, place it over medium-low heat, spray it with oil and when hot, pour in 1/3 cup of the prepared batter, spread it gently and cook for 5 to 7 minutes until the bottom turns golden brown; pour in more batter if there is a space on the pan.

7. Flip the pancake, continue cooking for 5 minutes, and when done, transfer pancake to a plate and then repeat with the remaining batter.

8. Serve pancakes with sliced bananas.

Nutrition: 190 Cal 14 g Fat 6 g Saturated Fat 8 g Carbohydrates 2 g Fiber 4 g Sugars 8 g Protein

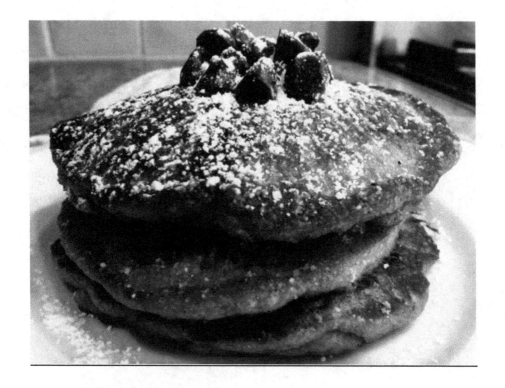

Berries and Banana Smoothie Bowl

Preparation Time: 5 minutes

Cooking Time: 0 minutes

Servings: 4

Ingredients:

For the Smoothie:

- 4 cups frozen mixed berries
- 4 small frozen banana, sliced
- 4 scoops of vanilla protein powder
- 12 tablespoons almond milk, unsweetened

For the Toppings:

- 4 tablespoons chia seeds
- 4 tablespoons shredded coconut, unsweetened
- 4 tablespoons hemp seeds
- ½ cup Granola
- Fresh strawberries, sliced, as needed

Directions:

1. Add mixed berries into a food processor along with banana and then pulse at low speed for 1 to 2 minutes until broken.

2. Add remaining ingredients for the smoothie and then pulse again for 1 minute at low speed until creamy, scraping the sides of the container frequently.

3. Distribute the smoothie among four bowls, then top with chia seeds, coconut, hemp seeds, granola, and strawberries and serve.

Nutrition: 214 Cal 2.5 g Fat 1.6 g Saturated Fat 47.5 g Carbohydrates 8.8 g Fiber 26 g Sugars 2.8 g Protein

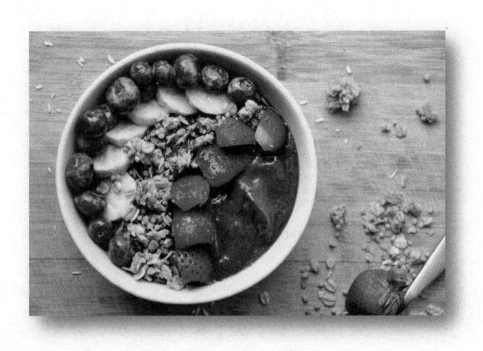

LUNCH

Loaded Kale Salad

Preparation Time: 10 minutes

Cooking Time: 30 minutes

Servings: 4

Ingredients:

- 1 ½ cup cooked quinoa

For The Vegetables:

- 1 whole beet, peeled, sliced

- 4 large carrots, peeled, chopped

- 1/2 teaspoon curry powder

- 1/8 teaspoon sea salt

- 2 tablespoons melted coconut oil

For The Dressing:

- ¼ teaspoon of sea salt

- 2 tablespoons maple syrup

- 3 tablespoons lemon juice

- 1/3 cup tahini

- 1/4 cup water

For the Salad:

- 1/2 cup sprouts

- 1 medium avocado, peeled, pitted, cubed

- 1/2 cup chopped cherry tomatoes

- 8 cups chopped kale

- 1/4 cup hemp seeds

Directions:

1. Switch on the oven, then set it to 375 degrees F and let it preheat.

2. Take a baking sheet, place beets and carrots on it, drizzle with oil, season with curry powder and salt, toss until coated, and then bake for 30 minutes until tender and golden brown.

3. Meanwhile, prepare the dressing and for this, take a small bowl, place all the ingredients in it and whisk until well combined, set aside until required.

4. Assemble the salad and for this, take a large salad bowl, place kale leaves in it, add remaining ingredients for the

salad along with roasted vegetables, drizzle with prepared dressing and toss until combined.

5. Serve straight away.

Nutrition: 472 Cal 22.8 g Fat 3.8 g Saturated Fat 58.7 g Carbohydrates 12.5 g Fiber 9.2 g Sugars 14.6 g Protein;

Tuna Salad

Preparation Time: 10 minutes

Cooking Time: 0 minutes

Servings: 4

Ingredients:

- 1/2 cup chopped celery

- 3 cups cooked chickpeas

- 1 tablespoon capers, chopped

- 2 tablespoons sweet pickle relish

- 1 tablespoon yellow mustard paste

- 2 tablespoons mayonnaise

Directions:

1. Take a medium bowl, place chickpeas in it, add mustard and mayonnaise and mash by using a fork until peas are broken.

2. Add remaining ingredients and stir until well combined.

3. Serve straight away.

Nutrition: 207 Cal 7 g Fat 1 g Saturated Fat 27 g Carbohydrates 8 g Fiber 1 g Sugars 9 g Protein

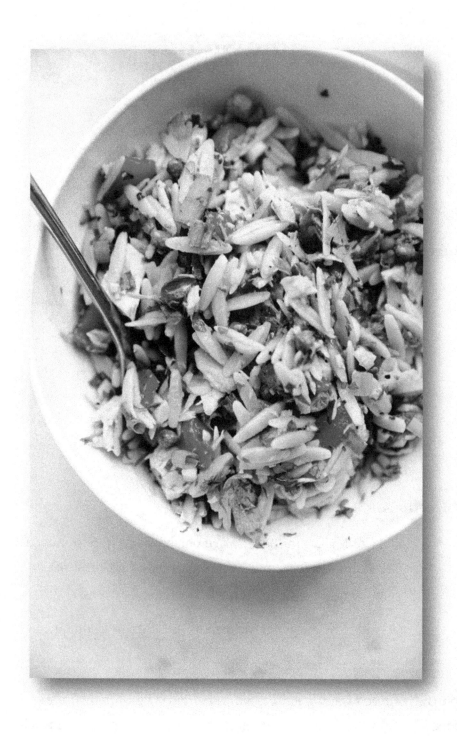

White Bean and Artichoke Sandwich

Preparation Time: 15 minutes

Cooking Time: 10 minutes

Servings: 4

Ingredients:

- 1 ¼ cooked white beans

- ½ cup cashew nuts

- 6 artichoke hearts, chopped

- ¼ cup sunflower seeds, hulled

- 1 clove of garlic, peeled

- ¼ teaspoon salt

- ¼ teaspoon ground black pepper

- 1 teaspoon dried rosemary

- 1 lemon, grated

- 6 tablespoons almond milk, unsweetened

- 8 pieces of rustic bread

Directions:

1. Soak cashew nuts in warm water for 10 minutes, then drain them and transfer into a food processor.

2. Add garlic, salt, black pepper, rosemary, lemon zest, and milk and then pulse for 2 minutes until smooth, scraping the sides of the container frequently.

3. Take a medium bowl, place beans in it, mash them by using a fork, then add sunflower seeds and artichokes and stir until mixed.

4. Pour in cashew nuts dressing, stir until coated, and taste to adjust seasoning.

5. Take a medium skillet pan, place it over medium heat, add bread slices, and cook for 3 minutes per side until toasted.

6. Spread white beans mixture on one side of four bread slices and then cover with the other four slices.

7. Serve straight away.

Nutrition: 220 Cal 8 g Fat 1 g Saturated Fat 28 g Carbohydrates 8 g Fiber 2 g Sugars 12 g Protein;

DINNER

Curried Apple

Preparation Time: 10 minutes

Cooking Time: 90 minutes

Servings: 4

Ingredients:

- 1 tablespoon fresh lemon juice

- ½ cup of water

- 2 apples, Fuji or Honeycrisp, cored and thinly sliced into rings

- 1 teaspoon curry powder

Directions:

1. Set the oven to 200F, take a rimmed baking sheet and line with parchment paper

2. Take a bowl and mix in lemon juice and water, add apples and soak for 2 minutes

3. Pat them dry and arrange in a single layer on your baking sheet, dust curry powder on top of apple slices

4. Bake for 45 minutes. After 45 minutes, turn the apples and bake for 45 minutes more

5. Let them cool for extra crispiness, serve and enjoy!

Nutrition: Calories: 240 Fat: 13g Carbohydrates: 20g Protein: 6g

Wild Rice and Millet Croquettes

Preparation Time: 5 minutes

Cooking Time: 20 minutes

Servings: 4

Ingredients:

- ¾ cooked millet
- ½ cup cooked wild rice
- 3 tablespoons extra virgin olive oil
- ¼ cup onion, minced
- 1 celery rib, finely minced
- ¼ cup carrot, shredded
- 1/3 cup all-purpose flour
- ¼ cup fresh parsley, chopped
- 2 teaspoons dried dill weed
- Salt and pepper to taste

Directions:

1. Add cooked millet and wild rice to a large-sized bowl, keep it to one side

2. Take a medium skillet and add 1 tablespoon of oil, place it over medium heat

3. Put onion, celery, and carrot and cook for at least 5 minutes

4. Add veggies and stir in flour, parsley, salt, pepper, and dill weed

5. Mix well and transfer to the fridge, let it sit for 20 minutes

6. Use hands to shape mixture into small patties, take a large skillet and place it over medium heat

7. Add 2 tablespoons of oil and let it heat up

8. Add croquettes and cook for 8 minutes in total until golden brown

9. Serve and enjoy!

Nutrition: Calories: 250 Fat: 9g Carbohydrates: 33g Protein: 9g

Grilled Eggplant Steaks

Preparation Time: 10 minutes

Cooking Time: 10 minutes

Servings: 4

Ingredients:

- 4 Roma tomatoes, diced
- 8 ounces cashew cream
- 2 eggplants
- 1 tablespoon olive oil
- 1 cup parsley, chopped
- 1 cucumber, diced
- Salt and pepper to taste

Directions:

1. Slice eggplants into three thick steaks, drizzle with oil, and season with salt and pepper

2. Grill in a pan for 4 minutes per side

3. Top with remaining ingredients

4. Serve and enjoy!

Nutrition: Calories: 86 Fat: 7g Carbohydrates: 12g Protein: 8g

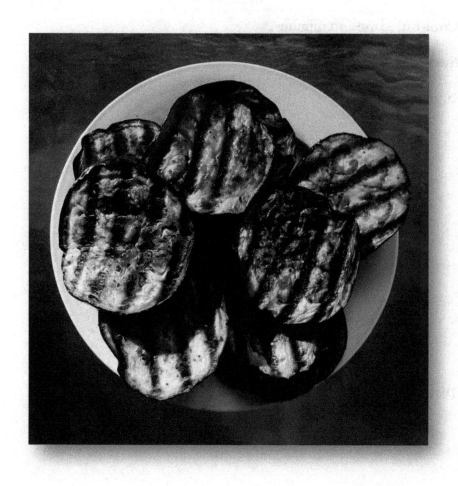

Steamed Cauliflower

Preparation Time: 5 minutes

Cooking Time: 10 minutes

Servings: 6

Ingredients:

- 1 large head cauliflower
- 1 cup water
- ½ teaspoon salt
- 1 teaspoon red pepper flakes (optional)

Directions:

1. Remove any leaves from the cauliflower, and cut it into florets.

2. In a large saucepan, bring the water to a boil. Place a steamer basket over the water, and add the florets and salt. Cover and steam for 5 to 7 minutes, until tender.

3. In a large bowl, toss the cauliflower with the red pepper flakes (if using). Transfer the florets to a large airtight container or 6 single-serving containers. Let cool before sealing the lids.

Nutrition: Calories: 35Fat: 0gProtein: 3gCarbohydrates: 7gFiber: 4gSugar: 4gSodium: 236mg

Cajun Sweet Potatoes

Preparation Time: 5 minutes

Cooking Time: 30 minutes

Servings: 4

Ingredients:

- 2 pounds sweet potatoes

- 2 teaspoons extra-virgin olive oil

- ½ teaspoon ground cayenne pepper

- ½ teaspoon smoked paprika

- ½ teaspoon dried oregano

- ½ teaspoon dried thyme

- ½ teaspoon garlic powder

- ½ teaspoon salt (optional)

Directions:

1. Preheat the oven to 400°F. Line a baking sheet with parchment paper.

2. Wash the potatoes, pat dry, and cut into ¾-inch cubes. Transfer to a large bowl, and pour the olive oil over the potatoes.

31

3. In a small bowl, combine the cayenne, paprika, oregano, thyme, and garlic powder. Sprinkle the spices over the potatoes and combine until the potatoes are well coated. Spread the potatoes on the prepared baking sheet in a single layer. Season with the salt (if using). Roast for 30 minutes, stirring the potatoes after 15 minutes.

4. Divide the potatoes evenly among 4 single-serving containers. Let cool completely before sealing.

Nutrition: Calories: 219Fat: 3gProtein: 4gCarbohydrates: 46gFiber: 7gSugar: 9gSodium: 125mg

Smoky Coleslaw

Preparation Time: 10 minutes

Cooking Time: 0 minute

Servings: 6

Ingredients:

- 1-pound shredded cabbage

- 1/3 cup vegan mayonnaise

- ¼ cup unseasoned rice vinegar

- 3 tablespoons plain vegan yogurt or plain soymilk

- 1 tablespoon vegan sugar

- ½ teaspoon salt

- ¼ teaspoon freshly ground black pepper

- ¼ teaspoon smoked paprika

- ¼ teaspoon chipotle powder

Directions:

1. Put the shredded cabbage in a large bowl. In a medium bowl, whisk the mayonnaise, vinegar, yogurt, sugar, salt, pepper, paprika, and chipotle powder.

2. Pour over the cabbage, and mix with a spoon or spatula and until the cabbage shreds are coated. Divide the coleslaw evenly among 6 single-serving containers. Seal the lids.

Nutrition: Calories: 73Fat: 4gProtein: 1gCarbohydrates: 8gFiber: 2gSugar: 5gSodium: 283mg

Mediterranean Hummus Pizza

Preparation Time: 10 minutes

Cooking Time: 30 minutes

Servings: 2 pizzas

Ingredients:

- ½ zucchini, thinly sliced

- ½ red onion, thinly sliced

- 1 cup cherry tomatoes, halved

- 2 to 4 tablespoons pitted and chopped black olives

- Pinch sea salt

- Drizzle olive oil (optional)

- 2 prebaked pizza crusts

- ½ cup Classic Hummus

- 2 to 4 tablespoons Cheesy Sprinkle

Directions:

1. Preheat the oven to 400°F. Place the zucchini, onion, cherry tomatoes, and olives in a large bowl, sprinkle them with the sea salt, and toss them a bit. Drizzle with a bit of

olive oil (if using), to seal in the flavor and keep them from drying out in the oven.

2. Lay the two crusts out on a large baking sheet. Spread half the hummus on each crust, and top with the veggie mixture and some Cheesy Sprinkle. Pop the pizzas in the oven for 20 to 30 minutes, or until the veggies are soft.

Nutrition: Calories: 500; Total fat: 25gCarbs: 58gFiber: 12gProtein:

STIR-FRIED, GRILLED VEGETABLES

Crusty Grilled Corn

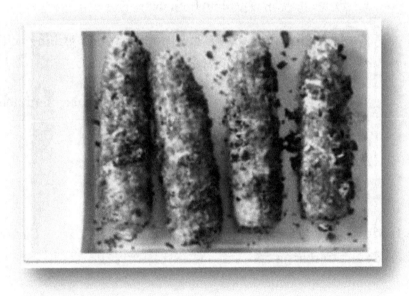

Preparation Time: 10 minutes

Cooking Time: 15 minutes

Servings: 4

Ingredients:

- 2 corn cobs

- 1/3 cup Vegenaise

- 1 small handful cilantro

- ½ cup breadcrumbs

- 1 teaspoon lemon juice

Directions:

1. Preheat the gas grill on high heat.

2. Add corn grill to the grill and continue grilling until it turns golden-brown on all sides.

3. Mix the Vegenaise, cilantro, breadcrumbs, and lemon juice in a bowl.

4. Add grilled corn cobs to the crumbs mixture.

5. Toss well then serve.

Nutrition: Calories: 253 Total Fat: 13g Protein: 31g Total Carbs: 3g Fiber: 0g Net Carbs: 3g

Grilled Carrots with Chickpea Salad

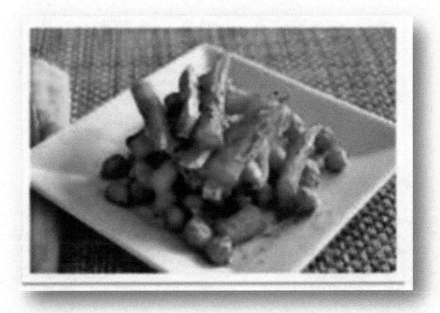

Preparation Time: 10 minutes

Cooking Time: 10 minutes

Servings: 8

Ingredients:

- Carrots

- 8 large carrots

- 1 tablespoon oil

- 1 ½ teaspoon salt

- 1 teaspoon dried oregano

- 1 teaspoon dried thyme

- 2 teaspoon paprika powder

- 1 ½ tablespoon soy sauce

- ½ cup of water

- Chickpea Salad

- 14 oz. canned chickpeas

- 3 medium pickles

- 1 small onion

- A big handful of lettuce

- 1 teaspoon apple cider vinegar

- ½ teaspoon dried oregano

- ½ teaspoon salt

- Ground black pepper, to taste

- ½ cup vegan cream

Directions:

1. Toss the carrots with all of its ingredients in a bowl.

2. Thread one carrot on a stick and place it on a plate.

3. Preheat the grill over high heat.

4. Grill the carrots for 2 minutes per side on the grill.

5. Toss the ingredients for the salad in a large salad bowl.

6. Slice grilled carrots and add them on top of the salad.

7. Serve fresh.

Nutrition: Calories: 661 Total Fat: 68g Carbs: 17g Net Carbs: 7g Fiber: 2g Protein: 4g

DIP AND SPREAD RECIPES

Black Bean and Corn Salsa from Red Gold

Preparation Time: 15 minutes

Cooking Time: 15 minutes

Servings: 25

Ingredients:

- 2 cans black beans, drained and rinsed

- 1 can whole kernel corn, drained

- 2 cans RED GOLD® Petite Diced Tomatoes & Green Chilies

- 1 can RED GOLD® Diced Tomatoes, drained

- 1/2 cup chopped green onions

- 2 tablespoon chopped fresh cilantro

- Salt and black pepper to taste

Directions:

1. Mix all ingredients to combine in a big bowl. Refrigerate to blend flavors for a few hours to overnight. Serve with chips or crackers.

Nutrition: Calories 65 Fat 3 Carbs 8 Protein 9

Avocado Bean Dip

Preparation Time: 15 minutes

Cooking Time: 15 minutes

Servings: 2

Ingredients:

- 1 medium ripe avocado, peeled and cubed
- 1/2 cup fresh cilantro leaves
- 3 tablespoon lime juice
- 1/2 teaspoon onion powder
- 1/2 teaspoon garlic powder
- 1/2 teaspoon chipotle hot pepper sauce
- 1/4 teaspoon salt
- 1/4 teaspoon ground cumin
- Baked tortilla chips

Directions:

1. Mix the first 9 ingredients in a food processor, then cover and blend until smooth. Serve along with chips.

Nutrition: Calories 85 Fat 4 Carbs 13 Protein 6

PASTA & NOODLES

Spicy Sweet Chili Veggie Noodles

Preparation Time: 10 minutes

Cooking Time: 7 minutes

Servings: 2

Ingredients:

- 1 head of broccoli, cut into bite sized florets

- 1 onion, finely sliced

- 1 tablespoon olive oil

- 1 courgette, halved

- 2 nests of whole-wheat noodles

- 150g mushrooms, sliced

- For Sauce

- 3 tablespoons soy sauce

- ¼ cup sweet chili sauce

- 1 teaspoon Sriracha

- 1 tablespoon peanut butter

- 2 tablespoons boiled water

- For Topping

- 2 teaspoons sesame seeds

- 2 teaspoons dried chili flakes

Directions:

1. Heat olive oil on medium heat in a saucepan and add onions.

2. Sauté for about 2 minutes and add broccoli, courgette and mushrooms.

3. Cook for about 5 minutes, stirring occasionally.

4. Whisk sweet chili sauce, soy sauce, Sriracha, water and peanut butter in a bowl.

5. Cook the noodles according to packet instructions and add to the vegetables.

6. Stir in the sauce and top with dried chili flakes and sesame seeds to serve.

Nutrition: Calories: 351 Total Fat: 27g Protein: 25g Total Carbs: 2g Fiber: 1g Net Carbs: 1g

SIDE DISHES

Coconut Cauliflower Mix

Preparation Time: 10 minutes

Cooking Time: 10 minutes

Servings: 6

Ingredients:

- 1 pound cauliflower florets

- 1 cup of water

- 1/4 cup of coconut milk

- 1 tablespoon coconut yogurt

- 1 teaspoon salt

- 1 teaspoon hot paprika

- 1 teaspoon Italian seasoning

- 1 tablespoon chives, chopped

Directions:

1. Place cauliflower and water in the instant pot. Add salt and close the lid.

2. Cook the vegetables on Manual mode for 10 minutes.

3. Then use quick pressure release.

4. Open the lid, drain water and mash the cauliflower.

5. Add the rest of the Ingredients, stir well and serve.

Nutrition: Calories: 211, Fat: 4.6, Fiber: 5.3, Carbs: 24.2, Protein: 3.9

Potato Mash

Preparation Time: 10 minutes

Cooking Time: 9 minutes

Servings: 6

Ingredients:

- 1 and 1/2 pounds white potatoes, peeled, chopped

- 1 teaspoon salt

- 1/2 teaspoon hot paprika

- 1 teaspoon dill, dried

- 1 tablespoon coconut butter

- 1 teaspoon ground black pepper

- 1 cup vegetable broth

- 1 tablespoon fresh parsley, chopped

Directions:

1. Put potatoes, salt, and vegetable broth in the instant pot.

2. Close the lid and set manual mode. Cook on High for 9 minutes.

3. Then make quick pressure release, strain the sweet potatoes and mash until smooth.

4. Add the rest of the Ingredients, stir well and serve.

Nutrition: Calories: 123, Fat: 4.3, Fiber: 2.2, Carbs: 11.4, Protein: 4.3

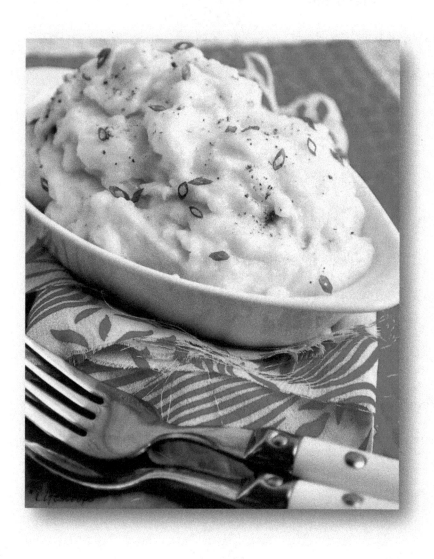

Red Cabbage and Carrots

Preparation Time: 10 minutes

Cooking Time: 7 minutes

Servings: 3

Ingredients:

- 1-pound red cabbage, shredded
- 2 carrots, peeled and grated
- 1 teaspoon turmeric powder
- 1 teaspoon coriander, ground
- 1 teaspoon black pepper
- 1 teaspoon salt
- 1/4 cup of coconut milk
- 3/4 cup almond milk
- 1/2 tablespoon chives, chopped

Directions:

1. In the instant pot, mix the cabbage with the carrots and the other Ingredients, toss and set manual mode (High pressure).

2. Cook the cabbage for 7 minutes. Then allow natural pressure release.

3. Transfer the meal into the serving bowls and cool down before serving.

Nutrition: Calories: 182, Fat: 5.1, Fiber: 3.4, Carbs: 12.3, Protein: 2.6

SOUP AND STEW

Cauliflower Spinach Soup

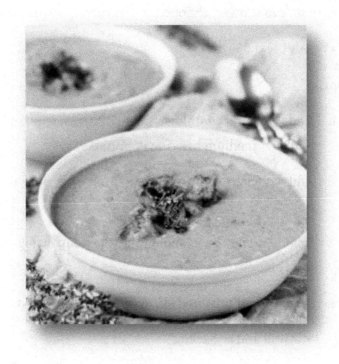

Preparation Time: 30 minutes

Cooking Time: 25 minutes

Servings: 5

Ingredients:

- 1/2 cup unsweetened coconut milk
- 5 oz. fresh spinach, chopped
- 5 watercress, chopped
- 8 cups vegetable stock
- 1 lb. cauliflower, chopped
- Salt

Directions:

1. Add stock and cauliflower in a large saucepan and bring to boil over medium heat for 15 minutes.
2. Add spinach and watercress and cook for another 10 minutes.
3. Remove from heat and puree the soup using a blender until smooth.
4. Add coconut milk and stir well. Season with salt.
5. Stir well and serve hot.

Nutrition: Calories: 271 kcal Fat: 3.7g Carbs: 54g Proteins: 6.5g

Creamy Squash Soup

Preparation Time: 10 minutes

Cooking Time: 25 minutes

Servings: 8

Ingredients:

- 3 cups butternut squash, chopped

- 1 ½ cups unsweetened coconut milk

- 1 tbsp. coconut oil

- 1 tsp dried onion flakes

- 1 tbsp. curry powder

- 4 cups water

- 1 garlic clove

- 1 tsp kosher salt

Directions:

1. Add squash, coconut oil, onion flakes, curry powder, water, garlic, and salt into a large saucepan. Bring to boil over high heat.

2. Turn heat to medium and simmer for 20 minutes.

3. Puree the soup using a blender until smooth. Return soup to the saucepan and stir in coconut milk and cook for 2 minutes.

4. Stir well and serve hot.

Nutrition: Calories: 271 kcal Fat: 3.7g Carbs: 54g Protein: 6.5g

Creamy Celery Soup

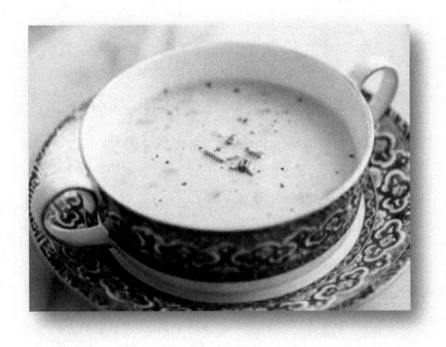

Preparation Time: 20 minutes

Cooking Time: 20 minutes

Servings: 4

Ingredients:

- 6 cups celery

- ½ tsp dill

- 2 cups water

- 1 cup coconut milk

- 1 onion, chopped

- Pinch of salt

Directions:

1. Add all ingredients into the electric pot and stir well.

2. Cover electric pot with the lid and select soup setting.

3. Release pressure using a quick release method than open the lid.

4. Puree the soup using an immersion blender until smooth and creamy.

5. Stir well and serve warm.

Nutrition: Calories: 159kcal Fat: 8.4g Carbs: 19.8g Proteins: 4.6g

Avocado Cucumber Soup

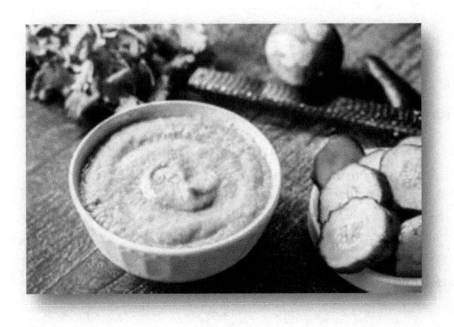

Preparation Time: 20 minutes

Cooking Time: 0 minutes

Servings: 3

Ingredients:

- 1 large cucumber, peeled and sliced

- ¾ cup water

- ¼ cup lemon juice

- 2 garlic cloves

- 6 green onion

- 2 avocados, pitted

- ½ tsp black pepper

- ½ tsp pink salt

Directions:

1. Add all ingredients into the blender and blend until smooth and creamy.

2. Place in refrigerator for 30 minutes.

3. Stir well and serve chilled.

Nutrition: Calories: 127 kcal Fat: 6.6g Carbs: 13g Protein: 0.7g

Garden Vegetable Stew

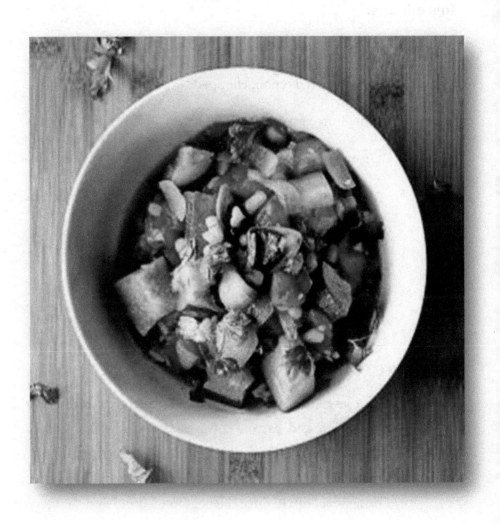

Preparation Time: 5 minutes

Cooking Time: 60 minutes

Servings: 4

Ingredients:

- 2 tablespoons olive oil

- 1 medium red onion, chopped

- 1 medium carrot, cut into 1/4-inch slices

- 1/2 cup dry white wine

- 3 medium new potatoes, unpeeled and cut into 1-inch pieces

- 1 medium red bell pepper, cut into 1/2-inch dice

- 11/2 cups vegetable broth

- 1 tablespoon minced fresh savory or 1 teaspoon dried

Directions:

1. In a large saucepan, heat the oil over medium heat. Add the onion and carrot, cover, and cook until softened, 7 minutes. Add the wine and cook, uncovered, for 5 minutes. Stir in the potatoes, bell pepper, and broth and bring to a boil. Reduce the heat to medium and simmer for 15 minutes.

2. Add the zucchini, yellow squash, and tomatoes. Season with salt and black pepper to taste, cover, and simmer until the vegetables are tender, 20 to 30 minutes. Stir in the corn, peas, basil, parsley, and savory. Taste, adjusting

seasonings if necessary. Simmer to blend flavors, about 10 minutes more. Serve immediately.

Nutrition: Calories: 219 kcal Fat: 4.5g Carbs: 38.2g Protein: 6.4g

Moroccan Vermicelli Vegetable Soup

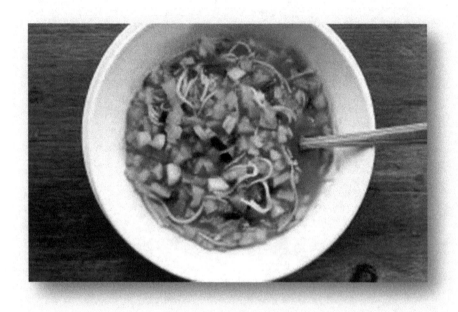

Preparation Time: 5 minutes

Cooking Time: 35 minutes

Servings: 4 to 6

Ingredients:

- 1 tablespoon olive oil

- 1 small onion, chopped

- 1 large carrot, chopped

- 1 celery rib, chopped

- 3 small zucchini, cut into 1/4-inch dice

- 1 (28-ounce) can diced tomatoes, drained

- 2 tablespoons tomato paste

- 11/2 cups cooked or 1 (15.5-ounce) can chickpeas, drained and rinsed

- 2 teaspoons smoked paprika

- 1 teaspoon ground cumin

- 1 teaspoon za'atar spice (optional)

- 1/4 teaspoon ground cayenne

- 6 cups vegetable broth, homemade (see light vegetable broth) or store-bought, or water

- Salt

- 4 ounces vermicelli

- 2 tablespoons minced fresh cilantro, for garnish

Directions:

1. In a large soup pot, heat the oil over medium heat. Add the onion, carrot, and celery. Cover and cook until softened, about 5 minutes. Stir in the zucchini, tomatoes,

tomato paste, chickpeas, paprika, cumin, za'atar, and cayenne.

2. Add the broth and salt to taste. Bring to a boil, then reduce heat to low and simmer, uncovered, until the vegetables are tender, about 30 minutes.

3. Shortly before serving, stir in the vermicelli and cook until the noodles are tender, about 5 minutes. Ladle the soup into bowls, garnish with cilantro, and serve.

Nutrition: Calories: 236 kcal Fat: 1.8g Carbs: 48.3g Protein: 7g

SMOOTHIES AND BEVERAGES

Cranberry and Banana Smoothie

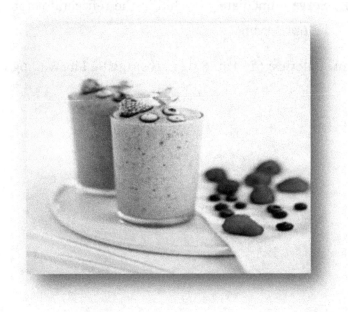

Preparation Time: 5 minutes

Cooking Time: 0 minutes

Servings: 4

- 1 cup frozen cranberries

- 1 large banana, peeled

- 4 Medjool dates, pitted and chopped

- 1½ cups unsweetened almond milk

Directions:

1. Add all the ingredients in a food processor, then process until the mixture is glossy and well mixed.

2. Serve immediately or chill in the refrigerator for an hour before serving.

Nutrition: Calories: 616 Fat: 8.0g Carbs: 132.8g Fiber: 14.6g Protein: 15.7g

Super Smoothie

Preparation Time: 5 minutes

Cooking Time: 0 minutes

Servings: 4

Ingredients:

- 1 banana, peeled
- 1 cup chopped mango
- 1 cup raspberries
- ¼ cup rolled oats
- 1 carrot, peeled
- 1 cup chopped fresh kale
- 2 tablespoons chopped fresh parsley
- 1 tablespoon flaxseeds
- 1 tablespoon grated fresh ginger
- ½ cup unsweetened soy milk
- 1 cup water

Directions:

1. Put all the ingredients in a food processor, then blitz until glossy and smooth.

2. Serve immediately or chill in the refrigerator for an hour before serving.

Nutrition: Calories: 550 Fat: 39.0g Carbs: 31.0g Fiber: 15.0g Protein: 13.0g

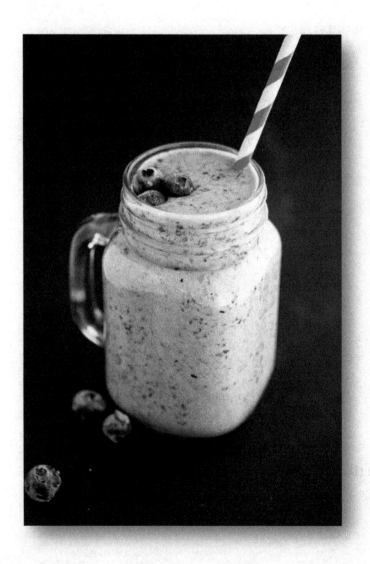

BREAD RECIPES

Sweet Rolls

Preparation Time: 2 hours

Cooking Time: 30 Minutes

Servings: 8

Ingredients:

- 2 tablespoons cane sugar

- 1 teaspoon rapid dry yeast

- 2 1/2 tablespoons warm water

- 1/2 cup pineapple juice, plus more for brushing tops of rolls

- 2 tablespoons coconut oil, melted

- 1 3/4 cups unbleached all-purpose flour, plus more for rolling out the dough

Directions:

1. In a small bowl, combine the sugar, yeast, and warm water. Stir gently and set aside for 10 minutes.

2. In another small bowl, combine 1/2 cup of pineapple juice and the coconut oil and stir.

3. Add the yeast mixture to the pineapple mixture and stir gently.

4. Add 1 3/4 cups of flour, and mix with your hands until well combined. The dough should not be too sticky. Knead in the bowl for 10 minutes, or until the dough is soft and smooth.

5. Place the dough in an oiled bowl, cover with a clean, damp towel, and place in a warm area for 1 hour to allow it to rise.

6. On a lightly floured surface, knead the dough, incorporating the flour from the surface. Break the dough into 8 equal pieces and form rolls.

7. Place the rolls on an oiled baking pan and allow to rise again for 30 to 40 minutes. Twenty minutes into this second rise, preheat the oven to 375 degree F.

8. Use a pastry brush to brush the tops of the rolls with pineapple juice.

9. Bake for 25 to 30 minutes or until golden brown.

Nutrition: Calories 115, Carbs 2.5g, Fat 11.5g, Protein 6.7g

Zero-Fat Carrot Pineapple Loaf

Preparation Time: 20 minutes

Cooking Time: 1.5 hours

Serving Size: 1 ounce (28.3g)

Ingredients:

- 2 ½ cups all-purpose flour

- ¾ cup of sugar

- ½ cup pineapples, crushed

- ½ cup carrots, grated

- ½ cup raisins

- Two teaspoons baking powder

- ½ teaspoon ground cinnamon

- ½ teaspoon salt

- ¼ teaspoon allspice

- ¼ teaspoon nutmeg

- ½ cup applesauce

- One tablespoon molasses

Direction:

1. Put first the wet ingredients into the bread pan before the dry ingredients.

2. Press the "Quick" or "Cake" mode of your bread machine.

3. Allow the machine to complete all cycles.

4. Take out the pan from the machine, but wait for another 10 minutes before transferring the bread into a wire rack.

5. Cooldown the bread before slicing.

Nutrition: Calories: 70 | Carbohydrates: 16g Fat: 0g | Protein: 1g

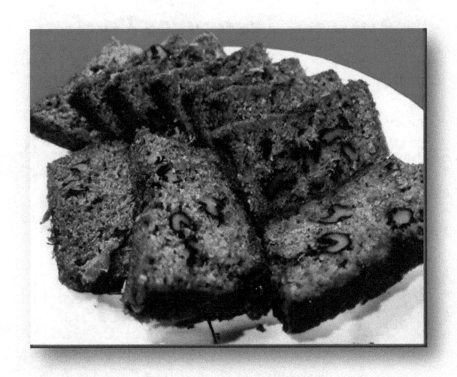

Autumn Treasures Loaf

Preparation Time: 15 minutes

Cooking Time: 1/5 hours

Serving Size: 1 ounce (28.3g)

Ingredients:

- 1 cup all-purpose flour

- ½ cup dried fruit, chopped

- ¼ cup pecans, chopped

- ¼ cup of sugar

- Two tablespoons baking powder

- One teaspoon salt

- ¼ teaspoon of baking soda

- ½ teaspoon ground nutmeg

- 1 cup apple juice

- ¼ cup of vegetable oil

- Three tablespoons aquafaba

- One teaspoon of vanilla extract

Direction:

1. Add all wet ingredients first to the bread pan before the dry ingredients.

2. Turn on the bread machine with the "Quick" or "Cake" setting.

3. Wait for all cycles to be finished.

4. Remove the bread pan from the machine.

5. After 10 minutes, transfer the bread from the pan into a wire rack.

6. Slice the bread only when it has completely cooled down.

Nutrition: Calories: 80 | Carbohydrates: 12g Fat: 3g | Protein: 1g

SAUCES, DRESSINGS, AND DIPS

Tahini BBQ Sauce

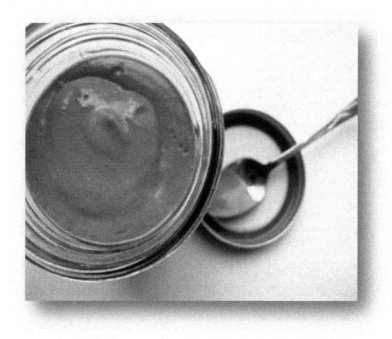

Preparation Time: 10 minutes

Cooking Time: 0 minutes

Servings: 4

Ingredients:

- ½ cup water

- ¼ cup red miso

- 3 cloves garlic, minced

- 1-inch (2.5 cm) piece ginger, peeled and minced

- 2 tablespoons rice vinegar

- 2 tablespoons tahini

- 2 tablespoons chili paste or chili sauce

- 1 tablespoon date sugar

- ½ teaspoon crushed red pepper (optional)

Directions:

1. Place all the ingredients in a food processor, and purée until thoroughly mixed and smooth. You can thin the sauce out by stirring in ½ cup of water, or keep it thick.

2. Transfer to the refrigerator to chill until ready to serve.

Nutrition: Calories: 206 Fat: 10.2g Carbs: 21.3g Protein: 7.2g Fiber: 4.4g

SALADS RECIPES

Cucumber Edamame Salad

Preparation Time: 5 minutes

Cooking Time: 8 minutes

Servings: 2

Ingredients:

- 3 tbsp. avocado oil

- 1 cup cucumber, sliced into thin rounds

- ½ cup fresh sugar snap peas, sliced or whole

- ½ cup fresh edamame

- ¼ cup radish, sliced

- 1 large Hass avocado, peeled, pitted, sliced

- 1 nori sheet, crumbled

- 2 tsp. roasted sesame seeds

- 1 tsp. salt

Directions:

1. Bring a medium-sized pot filled half way with water to a boil over medium-high heat.

2. Add the sugar snaps and cook them for about 2 minutes.

3. Take the pot off the heat, drain the excess water, transfer the sugar snaps to a medium-sized bowl and set aside for now.

4. Fill the pot with water again, add the teaspoon of salt and bring to a boil over medium-high heat.

5. Add the edamame to the pot and let them cook for about 6 minutes.

6. Take the pot off the heat, drain the excess water, transfer the soybeans to the bowl with sugar snaps and let them cool down for about 5 minutes.

7. Combine all ingredients, except the nori crumbs and roasted sesame seeds, in a medium-sized bowl.

8. Carefully stir, using a spoon, until all ingredients are evenly coated in oil.

9. Top the salad with the nori crumbs and roasted sesame seeds.

10. Transfer the bowl to the fridge and allow the salad to cool for at least 30 minutes.

11. Serve chilled and enjoy!

Nutrition: Calories 182 Total Fat 10.9g Saturated Fat 1.3g Cholesterol 0mg Sodium 1182mg Total Carbohydrate 14.2g Dietary

Fiber 5.4g Total Sugars 1.9g Protein 10.7g Vitamin D 0mcg, Calcium 181mg Iron 4mg Potassium 619mg

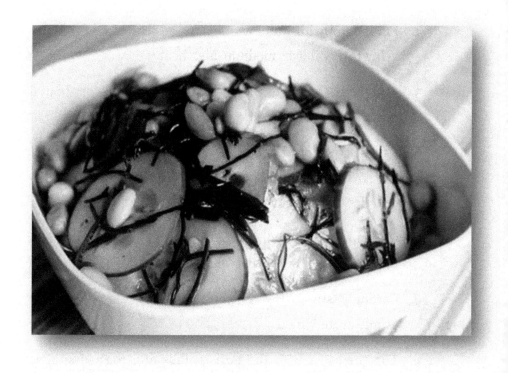

FRUIT SALAD RECIPES

Tropical Fruit Salad

Preparation Time: 10 Minutes

Cooking Time: 0 Minutes

Servings: 2

Ingredients:

- Lime juice, one tablespoon

- Kiwi, two

- Dragon fruit, one half of one

- Strawberries, twelve

- Mango, one half of one

Directions:

1. Peel the fruits and chop them into bite-sized pieces. Dump all of the fruit chunks into a large-sized mixing bowl.

2. Drizzle the lime juice over the fruit and toss the fruit gently to coat all of the pieces with the juice. Serve immediately

Nutrition: Calories: 154 Protein: 2g Fat: 1g Carbs: 37g

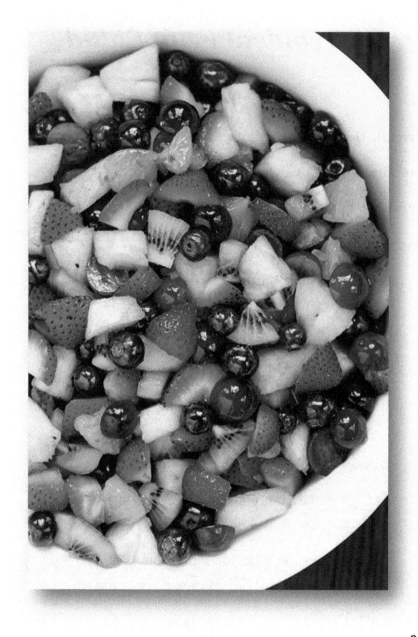

ENTRÉES

Veggie Hummus Wraps

Preparation Time: 10 minutes

Cooking Time: 6 minutes

Servings: 2

Ingredients:

- Zucchini, peeled, sliced lengthwise into .25-inch-thick strips – 1

- Sea salt - .5 teaspoon

- Tomato, sliced – 1

- Kale, chopped – 1 cup

- Red onion, sliced - .125 cup

- Avocado, sliced – 1

- Olive oil – 1 tablespoon

- Black pepper, ground - .25 teaspoon

- Apple cider vinegar – 2 teaspoons

- Water – 1 tablespoon

- Hummus - .25 cup

- Whole-wheat tortillas, large – 2

Directions:

1. Heat a large non-stick skillet or grill pan on the stove over medium heat. Meanwhile, coat the sliced zucchini with the olive oil, ground black pepper, and sea salt.

2. Place the seasoned zucchini on the preheated pan and let it cook on the first side for three minutes, flip it over, and cook for an additional two minutes. Remove the zucchini from the heat of the stove and set it aside.

3. Set the whole-wheat tortillas in the hot pan and allow them to toast for a minute. You want the tortillas to be lightly toasted, warm, and easy to wrap without tearing.

4. Combine the apple cider vinegar and water, then toss the avocado in the mixture. This will help prevent the avocado from browning. Drain off any excess liquid.

5. Divide the ingredients in half, so that you can fill both tortillas with an even amount of ingredients. To prepare spread the hummus down the center of the warm tortilla, top with the zucchini, tomato, red onion, kale, and avocado.

6. Wrap in the ends of the tortillas and then tightly wrap the sides around the filling. By folding it this way, you will

prevent the filling from falling out. Serve immediately or store in the fridge until lunchtime.

Nutrition: Number of Calories in Individual **Servings:** 438 Protein Grams: 9 Fat Grams: 28 Total Carbohydrates Grams: 40 Net Carbohydrates Grams: 36

GRAINS AND BEANS

Indian Lentil Dahl

Preparation Time: 10 minutes

Cooking Time: 25 minutes

Servings: 6

Ingredients:

- 3 cup cooked basmati rice

- 2 tablespoons olive oil (optional)

- 6 garlic cloves, minced

- 2 yellow onions, finely diced

- 1-inch piece fresh ginger, minced

- 2 tomatoes, diced

- 2 tablespoons ground cumin

- 1 tablespoon ground coriander

- 1 tablespoon ground turmeric

- 1 tablespoon paprika

- 4 cups water

- 2 cups uncooked green lentils, rinsed

- 1 teaspoon salt (optional)

Directions:

1. In a large pot, heat the olive oil (if desired) over medium heat. Add the garlic, onions, and ginger. Cook for 3 minutes, or until onions are golden. Add the tomatoes and cook for 2 minutes more, stirring occasionally. Stir in the cumin, coriander, turmeric and paprika.

2. Add the water and lentils. Cover and bring to a boil over high heat. Once boiling, stir and reduce the heat to a simmer. Cook, covered, for 20 minutes, stirring every 5 minutes, or until the lentils are fully cooked and beginning to break down. Season with salt (if desired) and stir.

3. Divide the rice evenly among 6 meal prep containers. Add an equal portion of the dahl to each container. Let cool completely before putting on lids and refrigerating.

Nutrition: Calories: 432 Fat: 17.2g Carbs: 58.8g Protein: 10.9g Fiber: 8.9g

DRINKS

Hibiscus Tea

Preparation Time: 1 Minute

Cooking Time: 5 minutes

Servings: 2 servings

Ingredients:

- 1 tablespoon of raisins, diced

- 6 Almonds, raw and unsalted

- ½ teaspoon of hibiscus powder

- 2 cups of water

Directions:

1. Bring the water to a boil in a small saucepan, add in the hibiscus powder and raisins. Give it a good stir, cover and let simmer for a further two minutes.

2. Strain into a teapot and serve with a side helping of almonds.

Tips:

As an alternative to this tea, do not strain it and serve with the raisin pieces still swirling around in the teacup.

You could also serve this tea chilled for those hotter days.

Double or triple the recipe to provide you with iced-tea to enjoy during the week without having to make a fresh pot each time.

Nutrition: Calories 139 Carbohydrates: 2.7g Protein: 8.7g Fat: 10.3

Lemon and Rosemary Iced Tea

Preparation Time: 5 minutes

Cooking Time: 10 minutes

Servings: 4 servings

Ingredients:

- 4 cups of water

- 4 earl grey tea bags

- ¼ cup of sugar

- 2 lemons

- 1 sprig of rosemary

Directions:

1. Peel the two lemons and set the fruit aside.

2. In a medium saucepan, over medium heat combine the water, sugar, and lemon peels. Bring this to a boil.

3. Remove from the heat and place the rosemary and tea into the mixture. Cover the saucepan and steep for five minutes.

4. Add the juice of the two peeled lemons to the mixture, strain, chill, and serve.

Tips: Skip the sugar and use honey to taste.

Do not squeeze the tea bags as they can cause the tea to become bitter.

Nutrition: Calories 229 Carbs: 33.2g Protein: 31.1g Fat: 10.2g

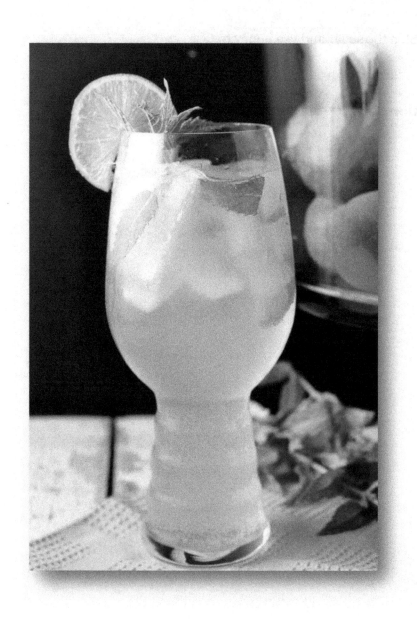

Lavender and Mint Iced Tea

Preparation Time: 5 minutes

Cooking Time: 10 minutes

Servings: 8 servings

Ingredients:

- 8 cups of water

- 1/3 cup of dried lavender buds

- ¼ cup of mint

Directions:

1. Add the mint and lavender to a pot and set this aside.

2. Add in eight cups of boiling water to the pot. Sweeten to taste, cover and let steep for ten minutes. Strain, chill, and serve.

Tips:

Use a sweetener of your choice when making this iced tea.

Add spirits to turn this iced tea into a summer cocktail.

Nutrition: Calories 266 Carbs: 9.3g Protein: 20.9g Fat: 16.1g

Energizing Ginger Detox Tonic

Preparation Time: 15 minutes

Cooking Time: 10 minutes

Servings:

Ingredients:

- 1/2 teaspoon of grated ginger, fresh

- 1 small lemon slice

- 1/8 teaspoon of cayenne pepper

- 1/8 teaspoon of ground turmeric

- 1/8 teaspoon of ground cinnamon

- 1 teaspoon of maple syrup

- 1 teaspoon of apple cider vinegar

- 2 cups of boiling water

Directions:

1. Pour the boiling water into a small saucepan, add and stir the ginger, then let it rest for 8 to 10 minutes, before covering the pan.

2. Pass the mixture through a strainer and into the liquid, add the cayenne pepper, turmeric, cinnamon and stir properly.

3. Add the maple syrup, vinegar, and lemon slice.

4. Add and stir an infused lemon and serve immediately.

Nutrition: Calories 443 Carbs: 9.7 g Protein: 62.8g Fat: 16.9g

DESERTS

Chocolate Avocado Ice Cream

Preparation Time: 1 hour and 10 minutes

Cooking Time: 0 minute

Servings: 2

Ingredients:

- 4.5 ounces avocado, peeled, pitted

- 1/2 cup cocoa powder, unsweetened

- 1 tablespoon vanilla extract, unsweetened

- 1/2 cup and 2 tablespoons maple syrup

- 13.5 ounces coconut milk, unsweetened

- 1/2 cup water

Directions:

1. Add avocado in a food processor along with milk and then pulse for 2 minutes until smooth.

2. Add remaining ingredients, blend until mixed, and then tip the pudding in a freezer-proof container.

3. Place the container in a freezer and chill for freeze for 4 hours until firm, whisking every 20 minutes after 1 hour.

4. Serve straight away.

Nutrition: Calories: 80.7 Cal Fat: 7.1 g Carbs: 6 g Protein: 0.6 g Fib er: 2 g

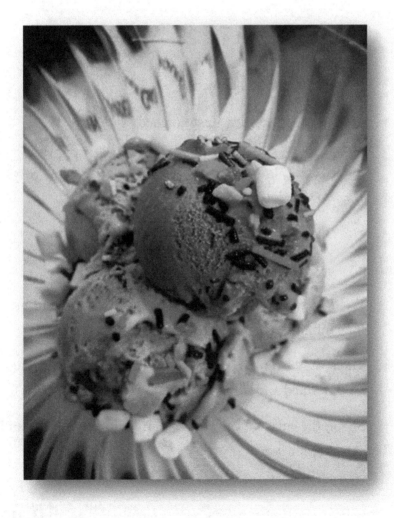

Chocolate Peanut Butter Energy Bites

Preparation Time: 1 hour and 5 minutes

Cooking Time: 0 minute

Servings: 4

Ingredients:

- 1/2 cup oats, old-fashioned

- 1/3 cup cocoa powder, unsweetened

- 1 cup dates, chopped

- 1/2 cup shredded coconut flakes, unsweetened

- 1/2 cup peanut butter

Directions:

1. Place oats in a food processor along with dates and pulse for 1 minute until the paste starts to come together.

2. Then add remaining ingredients, and blend until incorporated and very thick mixture comes together.

3. Shape the mixture into balls, refrigerate for 1 hour until set and then serve.

Nutrition: Calories: 88.6 Cal Fat: 5 g Carbs: 10 g Protein: 2.3 g Fiber: 1.6 g

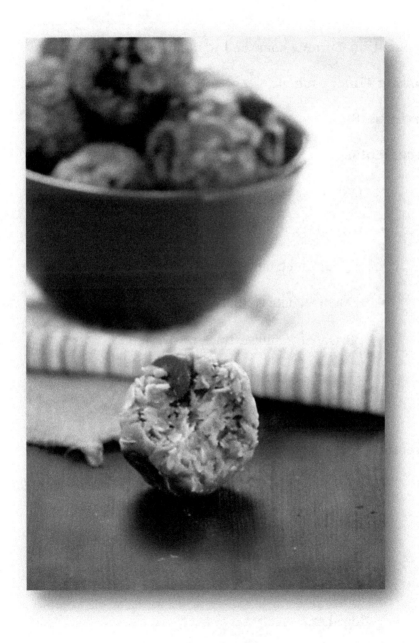

Cookie Dough Bites

Preparation Time: 4 hours and 10 minutes

Cooking Time: 0 minute

Servings: 18

Ingredients:

- 15 ounces cooked chickpeas

- 1/3 cup vegan chocolate chips

- 1/3 cup and 2 tablespoons peanut butter

- 8 Medjool dates pitted

- 1 teaspoon vanilla extract, unsweetened

- 2 tablespoons maple syrup

- 1 1/2 tablespoons almond milk, unsweetened

Directions:

1. Place chickpeas in a food processor along with dates, butter, and vanilla and then process for 2 minutes until smooth.

2. Add remaining ingredients, except for chocolate chips, and then pulse for 1 minute until blends and dough comes together.

3. Add chocolate chips, stir until just mixed, and then shape the mixture into 18 balls and refrigerate for 4 hours until firm.

4. Serve straight away

Nutrition: Calories: 200 Cal Fat: 9 g Carbs: 26 g Protein: 1 g Fiber: 0 g

Dark Chocolate Bars

Preparation Time: 1 hour and 10 minutes

Cooking Time: 2 minutes

Servings: 12

Ingredients:

- 1 cup cocoa powder, unsweetened
- 3 Tablespoons cacao nibs
- 1/8 teaspoon sea salt
- 2 Tablespoons maple syrup
- 1 1/4 cup chopped cocoa butter
- 1/2 teaspoons vanilla extract, unsweetened
- 2 Tablespoons coconut oil

Directions:

1. Take a heatproof bowl, add butter, oil, stir, and microwave for 90 to 120 seconds until melts, stirring every 30 seconds.

2. Sift cocoa powder over melted butter mixture, whisk well until combined, and then stir in maple syrup, vanilla, and salt until mixed.

3. Distribute the mixture evenly between twelve mini cupcake liners, top with cacao nibs, and freeze for 1 hour until set.

4. Serve straight away

Nutrition: Calories: 100 Cal Fat: 9 g Carbs: 8 g Protein: 2 g Fiber: 2 g

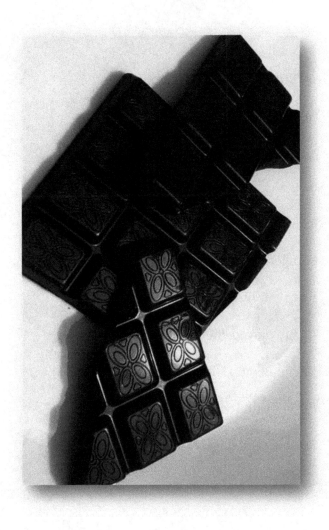

OTHER RECIPES

Lentil Potato Salad

Preparation Time: 10 minutes

Cooking Time: 25 minutes

Servings: 2

Ingredients:

- ½ cup beluga lentils

- 8 fingerling potatoes

- 1 cup thinly sliced scallions

- ¼ cup halved cherry tomatoes

- ¼ cup Lemon Vinaigrette

- Kosher salt, to taste

- Freshly ground black pepper, to taste

Directions:

1. Pour 2 cups of water to simmer in a small pot and add the lentils. Cover and simmer for 20 to 25 minutes, or until the lentils are tender. Drain and set aside to cool.

2. While the lentils are cooking, bring a medium pot of well-salted water to a boil and add the potatoes. Low heat to simmer and cook for about 15 minutes, or until the potatoes are tender. Drain. Once cool enough to handle, slice or halve the potatoes.

3. Place the lentils on a serving plate and top with the potatoes, scallions, and tomatoes. Drizzle with the vinaigrette and season with the salt and pepper.

Nutrition: Calories: 400 Fat: 26g Carbs: 39g Protein: 7g

Bok Choy–Asparagus Salad

Preparation Time: 20 minutes

Cooking Time: 0 minute

Servings: 4

Ingredients:

- 4 cups coarsely chopped baby bok Choy

- 1½ cups asparagus, trimmed and cut into 1½-inch lengths

- 1 cup cauliflower rice

- 1 cup strawberries, chopped into bite-size chunks

- 1 mango, peeled and diced

- ½ cup scallions, sliced into 1-inch lengths

- ¼ cup Lemon Vinaigrette

Directions:

1. In a large bowl, combine the bok choy, asparagus, cauliflower rice, strawberries, mango, and scallions. Drizzle with the vinaigrette and gently toss.

Nutrition: Calories: 210 Fat: 14g Carbs: 21g Protein: 3g

Vegan BBQ Tofu

Preparation Time: 10 minutes

Cooking Time: 40 minutes

Servings: 3

Ingredients:

- ¼ cup vegan BBQ sauce

- ¼ teaspoon pepper

- ¼ teaspoon garlic powder

- ¼ teaspoon salt

- 1 tablespoon grape seed oil

- 1 pack firm tofu

Directions:

1. Before you begin cooking your tofu, you will want to press it. Generally, this will take thirty to forty-five minutes. If possible, try to press the tofu overnight so that it is ready for you when you need it.

2. Once your tofu is ready, bring a saucepan over medium heat and allow it to warm up. As your saucepan is warming up, slice your tofu into small pieces. Put a 1 tablespoon of oil and spread your tofu across the pan. At

this point, season your tofu and cook for five minutes. Be sure to flip each piece of tofu until it is a nice golden-brown colour all over.

3. Finally, remove the tofu from the pan and cover it in BBQ sauce. This meal is excellent alone or with your favourite grain or vegetable.

Nutrition: Calories: 290, Fat: 64 g, Carbs: 25 g, Protein: 20 g

Mango Pineapple Hoisin Sauce

Preparation Time: 10 minutes

Cooking Time: 10 minutes

Servings: 2

Ingredients:

- 1 ½ cups fresh mango juice or pureed mango
- ⅔ cup vegan hoisin sauce
- 4 tablespoons brown rice vinegar
- 1 cup fresh pineapple juice
- ½ cup tamari or soy sauce
- 2 tablespoons Sriracha sauce

Directions:

1. Use a pan and heat oil over medium heat.
2. Add all the ingredients and stir constantly.
3. Simmer until the mixture thickens.

Nutrition: Calories: 125 Fat: 2 g Carbs: 8 g Protein: 4.3 g

CPSIA information can be obtained
at www.ICGtesting.com
Printed in the USA
LVHW011124090621
689684LV00011B/1391